medicare nj

2025 Edition – Navigating State and Federal Programs to Lower Your Medicare Expenses for New Jersey Residents

case publications

table of contents

📖 introduction: why this guide matters

If you're holding this book, chances are you're either feeling overwhelmed, frustrated, or just plain tired of trying to figure out how to afford Medicare. Maybe you've heard about things like PAAD, QMB, or NJ Save, but nobody's ever explained them in a way that actually makes sense. Maybe you've been told you "just miss" the income limit — and now you're wondering if there's anything out there for people like you.

You're not alone. And you're not crazy.

Medicare is complicated. And once you throw in all the state programs, assistance tiers, and paperwork, it can feel like a full-time job just to survive the system.

That's why I created this guide. Not to impress you with credentials. Not to bury you in technical language. But to give you a clear, step-by-step survival plan — specifically for New Jersey.

👋 who i am (and why you can trust this guide)

My name is **Danny**, and I've spent the last 9 years helping people navigate Medicare — not because I set out to become some kind of expert, but because I had to figure it out for someone who mattered to me: my mom.

When she turned 65, we got slammed with paperwork, robocalls, and more confusion than answers. So, I did what I had to do — I read the fine print, called the agencies, dug into every loophole, and made sure she got the coverage she deserved. Once her plan was set up, people around us started asking for help. And then their friends asked. And then their neighbors.

Nine years later, I've helped **thousands of New Jersey residents** understand and apply for these exact programs — from PAAD and QMB to Senior Gold, MLTSS, and more. I've seen clients go from paying $174/month for Medicare Part B to paying nothing — legally, ethically, and with peace of mind.

You won't see my name on the front cover — the name there is **Case Publications**, which I created in honor of my son. But I'm the one behind this book. I'm the guy who shows up when it's time to make sense of the system and fight for what you're owed.

This isn't theory. This is what I do. And this guide is written the way I talk to my real clients — with honesty, clarity, and no fluff. If you want to know exactly what programs exist, who qualifies, how to apply, and how to avoid the usual runaround, you're in the right place.

One last thing — the reason I've written this book with visual breaks, icons, and section dividers is because I know how **daunting** this kind of information can be. Honestly, most Medicare material out there is either confusing... or the next best sleep aid. I wanted to deliver this in a way that lets you **fully understand what you just read before moving on** — no racing through, no walls of text, no guessing. Just clarity. And maybe even a little enjoyment along the way.

what you'll learn in this book

This guide is all about helping you get real help, not just information. You'll find:

✅ A plain-English breakdown of every major New Jersey program that can lower your Medicare costs
✅ The exact income and asset limits — with no sugar-coating
✅ Who qualifies, what's covered, and how to apply
✅ A full walkthrough of the NJ Save application (with screenshots)
✅ A free printable PDF version you can download and follow along
✅ Real examples of how these programs helped my actual clients
✅ What to do if you don't qualify for anything — and how to stay prepared for next year

No sales pitch. No gimmicks. Just the help you were supposed to get years ago — finally explained the way it should've been.

🧭 why this matters (even if you think you don't qualify)

Every year, I meet people who think they're just over the limit or "not poor enough" to get help — and every year, we prove that wrong. Programs change. Income limits shift. Rules get adjusted. So, if you were denied before, that doesn't mean you'll be denied now.

Even if you don't get the big programs, there are still things you can do to lower costs, avoid penalties, or stay ready in case your situation changes. This book will show you those options too — because nobody should be navigating this system blind.

📌 before you start

Let me be real with you up front: this book won't solve Medicare. It's not going to erase all the red tape or make the state suddenly return your phone calls faster.

But it *will* do this:

It'll give you the clearest explanation of what's available in New Jersey — and how to take advantage of it.
It'll save you time.
It might save you money.
And it'll definitely help you feel less alone in the process.

So, take a breath. You've already done the hardest part by picking up this book.

Let's get started.

📖 chapter 1: what programs are out there?

If you've ever sat through a Medicare presentation or tried to make sense of the state's websites, you know what I mean when I say: it's a jungle out there. Everyone says, "There's help available," but nobody really explains *what kind of help*, *where to look*, or *if you even qualify*.

So, let's fix that.

Before we dive into applications, paperwork, and eligibility, I want to give you a **quick overview** of what New Jersey actually offers. You'll see that there isn't just one program — there's a **network of programs**, many of which can **stack together** to help you save on prescriptions, premiums, doctor visits, and even transportation.

what kind of help does new jersey offer?

Here are the **main categories of assistance** available to New Jersey residents on Medicare. Some are state programs, and some — like LIS — are federal. But the real power comes from **how they work together**.

✅ **Prescription Drug Help**

→ **PAAD** and **Senior Gold** reduce your out-of-pocket costs at the pharmacy.
→ **LIS (Low-Income Subsidy)**, also known as *Extra Help*, is a **federal** program that can lower your Part D premiums, eliminate your deductible, and cap your copays.
→ When combined, **PAAD + LIS** gives you even more protection. You'll pay **no deductible**, and your copays will often be lower than with either program alone — with steady, affordable pricing throughout the year.

✅ **Premium Help (Part B)**

→ **Medicare Savings Programs** (QMB, SLMB, QI) can pay your monthly Part B premium. Some also cover deductibles and copays depending on your income.

✅ **Long-Term Care Help**

→ **MLTSS** helps cover in-home care, assisted living, or nursing home expenses if you meet both financial and medical criteria.

✅ **Full Medicaid Coordination**

→ If you qualify for **NJ FamilyCare**, you may get additional benefits like dental, vision, and transportation layered on top of your Medicare coverage.

✅ **Utility Assistance**

→ **Lifeline** gives a $225 yearly credit toward your electric or gas bill, a year — freeing up money you can use elsewhere.

🛠️ so… how do you apply?

This part trips people up, because not all programs are handled the same way. But don't worry — here's how it breaks down:

📝 **For most New Jersey state programs**, like PAAD, Senior Gold, QMB/SLMB, and Lifeline, you'll use the **NJ Save application.** It's a single form that screens you for multiple programs at once.

🌐 **For LIS (Low-Income Subsidy)**, it's a little different — you apply through **Social Security** (either online, over the phone, or by mail). But here's the good news:

If you qualify for **QMB, SLMB, or full Medicaid**, you'll often be **automatically enrolled** into LIS. So, you might not need a separate application at all.

★ **Important:** Many people don't even realize they already have LIS because it gets applied behind the scenes. In Chapter 2, I'll show you how to confirm if you already have it — and how to apply if you don't.

Let's be real: the programs aren't the problem — it's how they're explained. Here's what usually trips people up:

- The **acronyms:** QMB, LIS, MLTSS, PDP... it's alphabet soup.
- The **income and asset rules**, which change every year and vary by program.
- The mix of **state and federal programs.** People assume it's all handled in one place, but in reality, LIS is federal, while PAAD and Senior Gold are state-run.

And the biggest myth?

"If I don't qualify for Medicaid, I don't qualify for anything."

Wrong.

You may not qualify for **full Medicaid**, but that doesn't mean you can't qualify for **other help** — like LIS, QMB, PAAD, or utility assistance.

In this book, I'll break it all down in a way that makes sense — and more importantly, show you **how to use these programs together** to actually reduce your out-of-pocket costs.

📌 what you'll see next

In the next chapter, we'll walk through the **NJ Save application** step by step — including what to fill out, what documents you'll need, and what to skip if it doesn't apply to you.

You'll also get:

- A printable checklist
- In-book screenshots
- A free downloadable PDF walkthrough
- And clear guidance on LIS and how to check if you already have it

No guessing. No red tape. Just the next step forward.

📘 chapter 2: how to apply for help without getting lost in the paperwork

If you've ever tried to apply for help with your Medicare costs before, you already know how it feels: confusing, frustrating, and more complicated than it needs to be. And if this is your first time? I'm going to make sure it goes a lot smoother.

The good news is: in New Jersey, most of the programs we talked about in Chapter 1 can be started using **just one application** — the **NJ Save** form.

This chapter will walk you through:

- What programs are included
- What documents you need to have ready
- A full breakdown of the online application (with screenshots)
- And how to avoid the mistakes that trip people up every year

We're going step by step — and by the end, you'll know exactly what to do and why it matters.

---

what is nj save?

NJ Save is a single application that screens New Jersey residents for several key Medicare-related assistance programs.

By filling it out once, you can be considered for:

✅ **PAAD (Pharmaceutical Assistance to the Aged and Disabled)**
✅ **Senior Gold**
✅ **Medicare Savings Programs (QMB, SLMB, QI)**
✅ **Lifeline Utility Assistance**
✅ Other potential Medicaid-related supports (like MLTSS, if applicable)

★ **Important:** NJ Save does **not** directly apply you for LIS (Low-Income Subsidy). That's a federal program run through Social Security. But if you qualify for QMB, SLMB, or Medicaid through NJ Save, you may be automatically enrolled into LIS anyway — more on that later in the chapter.

---

who should apply?

If you're a New Jersey resident and enrolled in Medicare, you should **absolutely** apply — even if:

- You've been denied before
- You think your income is a little too high
- You're not sure which program is the right on

Here's why:

NJ Save is a "smart" application. It uses your information to match you with the programs you *do* qualify for — even if you don't know the names of those programs yourself.

I tell clients this all the time:

"Let the system tell you no. Don't talk yourself out of trying."

---

what you'll need to apply

Before you jump into the application, it helps to gather your paperwork. Most of it is simple — you probably already have it in your kitchen drawer.

Here's what to have ready:

✅ **Medicare card** (you'll need the number and effective dates)
✅ **Social Security award letter** or proof of monthly income

☑ **Pension or other retirement income** (if you have any)
☑ **Bank statements or investment info** (for asset limits on certain programs)
☑ **Proof of NJ residency** (like a utility bill or driver's license)
☑ **If married:** income info for your spouse too, even if they're not on Medicare

★ **Important:** Keep these documents **handy** and **only submit them** with your application. Over-submitting can actually hurt your chances — let the state tell you what they want. There have been plenty of cases where clients were approved **right away** without sending a single supporting document — just the application itself. If your only income is from Social Security, and you don't have savings or retirement accounts, the application is pretty straightforward. But even if you have a few assets, don't panic — some programs (like PAAD and Senior Gold) **don't count assets at all.**

---

how to access the application

The NJ Save application can be completed online at:

https://njdoas-ua.force.com/njsave

You can also request a paper copy by calling:

📞 **1-800-792-9745** (NJ Department of Human Services)

I always recommend using the **online version** if you're comfortable — it's faster, cleaner, and you'll get a response sooner.

---

what the application looks like

The application is broken into simple sections:

1. **Basic Information**
   - Your name, address, contact info, Medicare number, and Social Security number
   - You'll be asked for marital status and date of birth
2. **Income Section**
   - This is where you list your monthly income (from Social Security, pensions, etc.)
   - They ask for the **gross amount** before deductions
3. **Assets Section**
   - You'll only fill this out if applying for programs that use asset limits (like QMB/SLMB)
   - This includes checking, savings, IRAs, stocks, or other accounts
4. **Expenses and Other Info**
   - You may be asked if you pay for health insurance, rent, or utilities — this is used to assess eligibility for certain programs

    - If you have a Medicare Advantage or Part D plan, list it here
5. **Signature and Submission**
    - You can sign digitally and submit immediately if online
    - If you're mailing a paper copy, don't forget to sign and date it

★ **Important:** Please refer to the **PDF walkthrough** for a complete, annotated version of this application. It gives you a step-by-step guide on what to fill out, what not to touch, and why it matters. Always remember — **less is more.** The goal is to give them exactly what they need, and nothing that could raise unnecessary questions.

🧠 what happens after you apply?

Once you submit your application, here's what to expect.

- If you applied online, you'll get a **confirmation number** immediately.
- Under normal conditions, you might hear back in 2–4 weeks.

But let's be honest — **2025 is not normal.**

★ **Important:** Due to higher income limits and a flood of new applicants, the NJ Save department is currently

severely backed up. It may take **up to 3 months** before you hear anything back. Do not panic — just be prepared to wait.

If the state **requests additional documentation**, you will receive a letter asking for it. This is critical:

You have **30 days** to respond to that letter.

If you miss that window, you'll have to **start the entire process over.**

Now, if you're approved right away — congrats. Here's what to look out for:

- On one of the pages in your approval packet, check the **bottom-right corner.**
- You'll find a **perforated card** that you can tear out:
  - A **bright yellow or gold card** means you've been approved for **PAAD**
  - A **white card with gold borders** means you've been approved for **Senior Gold**

These cards are real — and important. You'll need them at the pharmacy to get your copay discounts.

★ **Important:** The card might say it expires in 1 year, but don't let that confuse you. **PAAD and Senior Gold are valid for 2 years.**

At the end of the **first year**, the state will automatically mail you a **new card** with updated dates — no action needed.

Toward the end of the **second year**, you'll receive a renewal packet in the mail. That's your reminder to reapply if you still qualify.

As for the other programs (like QMB, SLMB, or Lifeline)?

Those approvals will arrive in **separate mailings** from either the state Medicaid office or Social Security, depending on the program.

---

how to check if you already have lis

LIS — also called Extra Help — is one of the most misunderstood benefits out there. Most people don't even realize they have it... until they see lower prescription copays or get told by the pharmacy that they "don't owe a deductible."

Here's how to check if it's already been applied:

✅ **Option 1: Review your Medicare Summary Notice (MSN)**

If you're receiving LIS, you'll often see language that says your **Part D premium is partially or fully paid**, or that your **copay has been reduced** under Extra Help.

✅ **Option 2: Call your Part D plan carrier**

Ask them: "Do I currently have Low-Income Subsidy/Extra Help applied to my account?"

They'll be able to tell you right away.

Option 3: If you have Medicare Advantage, call your insurance carrier

Ask them directly if you currently receive **LIS (Extra Help)** through your plan. Most carriers can tell you immediately if it's active on your file.

Option 4: Call Medicare directly – last option, options 1, 2, and 3 are the fastest way to

1-800-MEDICARE (1-800-633-4227)

They can confirm your LIS status, and if you don't have it, they can direct you to apply through Social Security.

★ **Important:** If you were approved for QMB, SLMB, or full Medicaid, you may already be enrolled in LIS automatically. But it's always worth double-checking — because if you're not getting it, you're likely overpaying for your medications.

---

if you need to reapply or were denied

Let's say you went through the whole process and got a denial letter — or worse, no response at all. Here's what to do.

Step 1: Double-check the reason

The denial letter will usually list a specific reason (e.g., income too high, missing documents, signature error).

Don't guess — read it carefully.

📌 **Step 2: Fix it and reapply**

If it's something small, like a document they didn't receive, **you can usually resubmit what they asked for without starting over.**

If your denial was based on income or assets, don't give up — **reapply next year**

These limits change **every January**, and one year's "no" can easily turn into a "yes" the following year — especially with inflation adjustments.

📌 **Step 3: Stay organized**

Keep a folder for:

- Your NJ Save confirmation number
- Any letters or requests from the state
- Copies of your submitted application
- Notes about when you called or followed up

You'd be surprised how many people get approved **months later** because they had the paper trail ready to go.

📥 how to download the full walkthrough pdf

This chapter has walked you through the process, but if you're the type who likes to **see things visually**, I've built something extra to help you out:

★ **Important:**

You can download a **free printable PDF** that shows every page of the NJ Save application, NJ Medicaid, and Extra Help/LIS — with arrows, screenshots, and instructions on what to fill in, and what to skip.

It's perfect if you want to preview the application or print it out to follow along.

https://casepub.gumroad.com/l/wzevud - NJSAVE APPLICATION GUIDE
http://casepub.gumroad.com/l/pvanbe - MEDICAID APPLICATION GUIDE
http://casepub.gumroad.com/l/jptlio - EXTRA HELP/LIS APPLICATION GUIDE

This guide is updated every year and built to make your life easier — because no one should have to guess their way through a government form. You can grab the latest version by creating a free Gumroad account. It's completely free and included with your book purchase. Once you download it, the step-by-step PDF will be sent straight to your email — no extra steps, no hassle.

---

final thoughts before we move on

This chapter may have felt like a lot, but if you take it one step at a time, you'll get through it.

Here's what I want you to remember:

- The NJ Save application covers **multiple programs** with one form
- You don't need to include all your documents upfront — only when asked
- Some programs may approve you automatically based on your answers
- If you were denied before, **try again** — rules change every year
- Once approved, **keep those cards** and letters in a safe place
- Use the tools in this book and the printable PDF to stay ahead of the game

You don't need to be an expert to get this right — you just need someone who's been through it to walk you through it.

That's what this book is for. And we're just getting started.

---

up next: real people, real savings

In the next chapter, I'm going to introduce you to a few real scenarios — people I've helped over the years — who went through this same process, found programs they didn't know they qualified for, and ended up saving big.

You'll see:

- How the system actually works in real life
- What success looks like for people in different income brackets
- And how one application can make thousands of dollars' worth of difference

Let's move from theory... to reality.

📘 chapter 3: real people, real savings

The biggest question I get — after we talk through all the programs — is this:

"Yeah, but does anyone actually *get* this stuff?"

And my answer is always the same:

Yes. All the time.

I've helped people save thousands, sometimes thousands, just by helping them fill out one form correctly. I've seen someone go from paying $500 a month in medications… to $14.20.

This chapter is where I show you what it really looks like when these programs work — and how people just like you got there. These are **real stories**, based on real New Jersey residents I've personally worked with. Names and a few small details have been changed to protect privacy, but the savings? The outcomes? All real.

👤 client a: the widow with the $174 surprise

Background:

Client A was 68, widowed, and living on just Social Security. When she came to me, she had just gotten her first Medicare statement showing a **$174.70 deduction** for Part B. She said, "I thought Medicare was free — what the hell is this?"

What we did:

After reviewing her income, I told her she qualified for **QMB**, one of the Medicare Savings Programs. That meant the state would cover her **Part B premium**, **any deductibles**, and **most copays** — all at no cost to her. We filed through NJ Save and got her approved in about 6 weeks.

Bonus benefit:

Because she qualified for QMB, she was **automatically enrolled in LIS (Extra Help)**. That lowered her drug copays too — from over $100/month down to $4–$9 for most meds.

Her reaction?

"Wait... I don't owe anything now? Just like that?"

She kept shaking her head like it was too good to be true. But it wasn't. It was just the system — finally working *for* her instead of against her.

client b: "too rich" for paad, but not out of options

Background:

Client B and his wife both had Medicare, but his income was **just over the PAAD limit.** He had heard about it through a friend but assumed he wouldn't qualify because they were "doing okay."

What we did:

After reviewing his numbers, I confirmed — yep, they were **over PAAD** by about $4,000 a year. But they weren't out of luck. I showed them **Senior Gold**, which kicks in at a higher income bracket.

How it helped:

Tony paid **$15** per prescription, and then the program covered **50% of the remaining cost.** It wasn't as generous as PAAD, but it still knocked their out-of-pocket costs in half.

They also hit their **out-of-pocket max** for the year — $2,000 for an individual or $3,000 for a couple. After that, Senior Gold picked up the rest.

★ **Important:** This is why it pays to look at **all** the programs — not just the "famous" ones. PAAD might get the spotlight, but **Senior Gold quietly helps thousands** of people every year who don't qualify for anything else.

👤 client c: caring for a disabled adult child

Background:

Client C was 73, on Medicare, and the full-time caregiver for her adult son with multiple disabilities. She handled all his medical paperwork, and when she found out he was aging into Medicare due to disability, she panicked.

What we did:

We reviewed her son's benefits. He was getting SSDI, had limited income, and qualified for both **QMB and MLTSS.**

- QMB took care of his premiums and copays
- MLTSS provided **home care, transportation**, and even helped her get a **personal care assistant** for a few hours each day

How it changed her life:

She cried during our third appointment. Not because she was overwhelmed this time — but because she finally had help.

"I didn't know you could get this much support if you weren't in a nursing home."

★ **Important:** Programs like **MLTSS** don't just pay for care — they give caregivers their life back. But they're complex, and the paperwork alone can make people give up before they start. That's why this book walks you through the process and shows you what to expect.

---

what these stories mean for you

You may have seen a little of yourself in these stories — or maybe not. Maybe your situation is different. That's okay. These programs weren't built for one type of person — they were built to **catch people who fall through the cracks.** People who worked hard, paid taxes, and now just want to make their Medicare work without going broke.

The truth is, most people who get help **never thought they'd qualify.**

They either assumed their income was too high, or that help was only for "poor people," or they were just overwhelmed and gave up. I'm here to tell you — if there's even a **chance** you qualify, it's worth applying. Because these programs aren't a handout. They're a **payback.**

You've already earned this help.

Now it's about making sure you get it.

★ **Important:** These aren't just financial wins — they're *life* wins. Less money going to prescriptions means more money for groceries. Fewer bills means fewer decisions you have to make under stress. A care program like MLTSS doesn't just support your loved one — it gives you **time back** to breathe, rest, and live.

---

what comes next

In the next chapter, we'll break down what to do **if you didn't qualify** for anything — or if you got denied and feel like you're out of options.

There are still strategies, tools, and lesser-known paths to lighten the load — even if the "big programs," said no.

Don't count yourself out. Let's explore what else is out there.

📔 chapter 4: what if i don't qualify for anything?

Let's say you went through the whole application process. You filled out NJ Save. You waited. You got the letter. And it said:

Denied.

Now what?

You're not alone. And you're not out of luck.

In fact, this chapter is **specifically for you.** Because even if you don't qualify for one of the "main" state programs right now, there are still ways to save money, avoid penalties, and prepare to try again — without starting from scratch.

I've helped thousands of people in this exact situation, and many of them *did* qualify the following year. Some found alternative resources they never knew existed. And almost all of them said the same thing:

"I wish someone had just told me what to do next."

So, let's talk about what to do next.

🔁 first — reapply next year (seriously)

Income and asset limits change every January.

So even if you're just $200 over the limit today, you might be under it next time around.

Here's what I tell my clients:

Don't take this year's "no" personally. These programs move.

Let's put a reminder in the calendar to reapply **January 1st** every year.

★ **Important:** PAAD, Senior Gold, and QMB/SLMB have adjusted their income limits multiple times over the past few years — sometimes by thousands. One denial doesn't mean you're out forever. It just means **not right now.**

💊 prescription discount options (without state help)

If your biggest cost is medication, and you didn't get approved for PAAD, LIS, or any state program, there are still ways to reduce your drug costs without insurance.

Here's what I recommend:

✅ **GoodRx** – Print or text yourself free coupons for most brand-name and generic medications.

✅ **SingleCare** – Similar to GoodRx, and sometimes cheaper depending on the pharmacy.

✅ **CostPlus Drugs** – Mark Cuban's online pharmacy offering hundreds of medications at wholesale prices plus a flat markup and small fee.

✅ **Blink Health** – Another reliable pharmacy discount tool you can use instead of your Part D plan if the out-of-pocket is lower.

★ **Important:** These tools work **even if you have insurance** — just don't run your Part D card at the pharmacy. Show them the coupon instead and ask which price is lower.

You might be shocked how often the discount card beats your insurance price.

👵 other local & nonprofit resources to explore

Depending on where you live in New Jersey, there may be **county-level** or **nonprofit** resources that offer relief for older adults — especially those with fixed incomes or caregiving responsibilities.

Here are a few to check:

- **County Aging & Disability Resource Connection (ADRC)**

They often have grant programs for things like meal delivery, utility relief, transportation, and even home modifications.

www.state.nj.us/humanservices/doas/home/adrc.html

- **Hospital Financial Assistance Programs**

Every hospital is required to offer a charity care or discount program for low-income patients — even if you have Medicare.

- **Catholic Charities, Jewish Family Services, and other faith-based groups**

These organizations often help with everything from utility shut-off prevention to short-term food stipends. And they don't care what religion you are.

- **SNAP (food assistance)**

Many seniors think they won't qualify — but if your only income is Social Security, **you might.**

Apply here: www.nj.gov/humanservices/njsnap

★ **Important:** None of these programs are advertised like Medicare Advantage plans or Part D. You have to go looking — but they're out there, and they *do* help people stay afloat.

---

how to protect yourself going forward

Just because you didn't get approved this year doesn't mean you're powerless. The best way to turn a future "maybe" into a "yes" is to stay prepared.

Here's how to stay ahead of the game — even if you're not getting help right now.

---

1. keep a medicare binder or folder

This doesn't need to be fancy. Just one place where you store:

- Your NJ Save application confirmation
- Copies of denial or approval letters
- Medicare card and insurance details
- Bank statements, Social Security award letters, and any supporting docs you used

★ **Important:** I've had clients reapply the next year with **zero stress** just because they kept a folder. You'll thank yourself later.

📅 2. mark your reapply date every january

Don't wait for the state to tell you it's time. Be the one who stays ahead of the deadline. I always tell clients:

"January 1st is your personal Medicare New Year."

Even if the limits haven't been announced yet, you can start gathering updated income documents and checking your numbers. The earlier you get in the system, the sooner you can get approved — especially with the current state processing delays.

🔁 3. talk to a licensed medicare broker every year

Even if you don't qualify for assistance, you still have choices. A broker can help you:

- Review Medicare Advantage plans that offer **Part B givebacks**
- Switch drug plans to lower out-of-pocket costs
- Find plans that cover your specific doctors and prescriptions

- Spot changes in your coverage that could cost you later

★ **Important:** You never pay a licensed broker directly — their services are free to you. The insurance companies pay them. So, you're getting professional help at no cost.

If you're not working with someone yet, that's okay. Just don't try to figure this all out on your own every year. The system was built to be complicated — that doesn't mean you have to suffer through it.

🤔 but what if i just... don't want to deal with it?

I get it. The paperwork. The phone calls. The waiting. The jargon.

It's a lot.

But here's the thing I always remind people of:

You're not doing this because it's fun. You're doing it because you deserve a break.

You've paid into the system. You've done your time. Now it's time to let it work for you.

Even if the state says no this year...

Even if the pharmacy won't budge on copays...

Even if you're tired of trying...

Keep applying. Keep learning. Keep asking questions.

Because the people who eventually win with Medicare are the ones who **don't give up.**

END final thought

Not qualifying right now doesn't make you a failure. It makes you someone who's paying attention.

You already did more than most people do — you took the time to learn what exists.

Now you know:

- Where to look
- What your options are
- And how to try again next year — smarter and stronger

That's not a loss. That's a setup for your next win.

🩶 can i ask you for one small favor?

If this book has helped you — even just a little — I want to ask you for something that costs nothing but makes a big difference.

Please consider leaving a quick review on Amazon.

You don't have to write a long story. Just a few honest words about what this guide did for you — whether it helped you apply for something, made you feel more confident, or just gave you some peace of mind.

When you leave a review, you're not just helping me.

You're helping the next person who's overwhelmed, confused, and wondering if there's anything out there for them. You're letting them know they're not alone — and that someone took the time to make it make sense.

That's what this book was always about.

You can leave a review by searching **"2025 Medicare Help in New Jersey" on Amazon** and scrolling down to the review section.

Thank you for being part of this work.

You matter more than you know.

— **Danny**

Case Publications

📔 frequently asked questions (faq)

You've made it through a lot of information. Now let's slow it down and answer the kinds of questions people don't always feel comfortable asking — or that never get a straight answer online.

💬 if i get approved for one program, does that mean i'm approved for all of them?

No — but applying once can screen you for many.

If you use the **NJ Save application**, it will check to see if you're eligible for PAAD, Senior Gold, QMB/SLMB, and Lifeline. But **MLTSS, NJ FamilyCare, and LIS (Extra Help)** are handled separately and may require a second application or follow-up.

That said, **some programs trigger others** automatically. For example:

- If you qualify for QMB, you'll likely be auto-enrolled in LIS.
- If you get Medicaid, you'll also qualify for QMB and Part D help.

So, while approval for one doesn't guarantee approval for all, **it opens doors.**

💬 can i still apply if i'm just barely over the income limit?

Yes — and you should.

I always tell people: "**Let the system tell you no. Don't tell yourself no first.**"

Every year the limits change, and in 2025, many of them **went up.** If you were denied last year, you might qualify now. And even if you're just over, some programs (like Senior Gold) were built *specifically* for people who don't qualify for the others.

Apply. Worst case, they say no. Best case, you save hundreds.

💬 will getting help from paad or qmb affect my social security check?

No.

These are **non-taxable, non-cash benefits.** They won't reduce your Social Security check, and they don't get counted as "income" by IRS or benefit agencies.

In fact, some people see their Social Security check **go up** after qualifying — because programs like QMB pay your Part B premium, which is usually deducted from your check.

💬 i already have a medicare advantage plan. can i still apply for these programs?

Yes.

In fact, most of the people I help **already have Advantage plans.**

Programs like PAAD, QMB, and LIS work **alongside** your Advantage plan — they don't replace it. You may still have to stay in-network or follow plan rules, but your out-of-pocket costs can drop significantly.

★ **Important:** If you qualify for something like QMB or Medicaid, **your plan options may expand.** You could switch into a D-SNP (Dual-Eligible Special Needs Plan) with richer benefits like transportation, dental, and even grocery cards.

💬 can i get both paad and lis?

Yes — and they work beautifully together.

- **LIS (Extra Help)** is a federal program that reduces your drug costs under Medicare Part D.
- **PAAD** is a state program that caps your copays, pays your deductible, and even helps with premiums.

When used together, most people pay **$0 deductible** and have copays as low as **$5 for generics** or **$7 for brand-name drugs** — sometimes even less.

💬 what if i'm in a giveback plan? can i still apply for qmb or paad?

Yes — but you may have to choose between them.

A giveback plan refunds part of your **Part B premium**, but **QMB pays the whole thing** (and more). So, if you get approved for QMB, your giveback **goes away**, but your premium is fully covered — and your deductibles and copays too.

PAAD works **with** any Advantage or drug plan, including givebacks. So, there's no conflict there.

Bottom line: **QMB > giveback**

If you qualify for QMB, it's almost always the better deal.

---

i applied before and never heard back. should i apply again?

Yes — especially in 2025.

Due to the income limit increases, the NJ Save office is severely backed up.

Some people have waited **2–3 months** for a response.

Here's what you should do:

- If it's been longer than 90 days, call 1-800-792-9745 and ask for a status update.
- If you got a letter asking for more documents, **you only have 30 days to respond.** Miss that window and you'll have to start over.

★ **Important:** Don't assume they denied you if you didn't get a response. Call first — mistakes happen all the time.

💬 can i get help if i live with family or have adult children in the home?

Yes.

What matters is **your income and your spouse's** — not your adult children or grandchildren.

So, if you live with family but they don't contribute financially, you can still qualify.

Just make sure not to accidentally list someone else's income on the application. That's a common mistake that can trigger a denial.

💬 i don't have a printer or scanner. can i still apply?

Yes.

You can apply **online** without printing anything. If you don't have a computer, go to your local library or senior center — many of them offer free computer help.

If you prefer paper, you can request a mailed application by calling NJ Save:

📞 1-800-792-9745

★ **Important:** You **do not** need to send documents with your application unless the state asks for them later.

---

can i help my parent or grandparent apply?

Yes — and please do.

Many people never apply because they're intimidated by the paperwork or don't understand the questions.

You can fill out the NJ Save form **on their behalf** as long as you have their info.

If you're acting as their representative (like power of attorney or legal guardian), you may need to submit proof if the state requests it — but you don't need that to get started.

---

do i have to reapply every year?

Not always.

- **PAAD and Senior Gold** are valid for **2 years**, even if the card says 1. The state will automatically send a **new card after year one**, and a **renewal packet after year two.**

- **QMB/SLMB** and Medicaid programs usually require re-verification **every year**
- **LIS** can carry over, but you may get a **reassessment letter** asking for income updates

★ **Important:** Even if you don't get a renewal letter — reapply every **January 1st** just to be safe.

💬 what happens if my income goes up?

It depends.

If you're already approved and your income increases slightly, you may still qualify for:

- A different tier (like switching from QMB to SLMB)
- A program like Senior Gold instead of PAAD
- Or nothing at all — but you can still reapply the next year

If your income jumps a lot — from retirement, pension, or rental income — notify the program if you're asked to verify.

Don't guess — always reapply and let the system tell you yes or no.

📘 coming up next: the appendix

In the next section, you'll find a set of **quick-reference program sheets** you can print, photocopy, or hand to a friend.

Each one gives you the basics: income limits, benefits, and where to apply.

Because when you finally get that approval letter — you'll want to share the good news with someone else.

📘 appendix: program quick reference sheets

These quick-reference pages are designed for **copying, printing, or handing off to someone else** who needs help. Each sheet gives you the key info — no fluff, just facts.

✅ paad (pharmaceutical assistance to the aged and disabled)

Who It Helps:

- NJ residents age 65+ or receiving SSDI
- Enrolled in Medicare Part D (either stand-alone or through Advantage)

What It Covers:

- Caps drug copays at **$5 (generics)** and **$7 (brand-name)**
- Pays Part D annual deductible
- Pays up to **$48/month toward Part D premium &**

Medicare Advantage plan premiums (or late enrollment penalty — **whichever is less of the 3**)

- Includes discounts at the DMV for vehicle registration

Income Limits (2025):

- Single: **$53,446/year**
- Married: **$60,690/year**

Assets:

- **Not counted**

Where to Apply:

- ✅ Apply through NJ Save
- 🌐 https://njdoas-ua.force.com/njsave
- 📞 1-800-792-9745

✅ senior gold

Who It Helps:

- NJ residents 65+ or on SSDI
- Over the PAAD income limit but still under extended threshold

What It Covers:

- Copays: **$15 plus 50% of remaining cost**
- Out-of-pocket max: **$2,000/year (single)** or **$3,000/year (couple)**
- After reaching the cap, meds are free

Income Limits (2025):

- Single: **$53,446–$63,446**
- Married: **$60,690–$70,690**

Assets:

- **Not counted**

Where to Apply:

- ✅ Apply through NJ Save
- 🌐 https://njdoas-ua.force.com/njsave
- 📞 1-800-792-9745

✅ medicare savings programs (qmb, slmb, qi)

Who It Helps:

- Medicare enrollees with limited income
- Pays Part B premium, copays, or both depending on income

What It Covers:

Program	Pays Part B Premium	Covers Copays/Deductibles	LIS Auto-Enrollment
QMB	✅ Yes	✅ Yes	✅ Yes
SLMB	✅ Yes	❌ No	✅ Yes
QI	✅ Yes	❌ No	✅ Yes

Income Limits (2025):

Program	Single Income Limit	Married Income Limit	Asset Limit (Single)	Asset Limit (Married)
QMB	≤ $1,325/month	≤ $1,783/month	$9,660	$14,470
SLMB	≤ $1,585/month	≤ $2,135/month	$9,660	$14,470
QI	≤ $1,781/month	≤ $2,400/month	$9,660	$14,470

Asset Limits:

- Single: **$9,660**
- Married: **$14,470**

Where to Apply:

- ✅ Apply through NJ Save
- 🌐 https://njdoas-ua.force.com/njsave
- 📞 1-800-792-9745

✅ lifeline utility assistance

Who It Helps:

- NJ residents 65+ or on SSDI
- Must be enrolled in PAAD, Medicaid, SSI, SNAP, or subsidized housing

What It Covers:

- **$225 annual credit** toward electric or gas bills
- **$225** will be **sent directly to your utility company.** It will show as a credit on your bill.
- Helps free up budget for other medical expenses

Income:

- Follows the PAAD guidelines
- Must qualify for a primary program like PAAD or Medicaid

Assets:

- **Not counted**

Where to Apply:

- ☑️ Apply through NJ Save
- 🌐 https://njdoas-ua.force.com/njsave
- 📞 1-800-792-9745

☑️ managed long term services and supports (mltss)

Who It Helps:

- NJ residents age 65+ or disabled
- Must require a **nursing home level of care** (even if staying at home)
- Common for those needing **home care, assisted living**, or **long-term supports**

What It Covers:

- Home health aides and personal care
- Medical day care, transportation, meals
- Assisted living and nursing facility costs
- Support for caregivers
- Includes coordination with Medicare and Medicaid

Income Limit (2025):

- Single: **$2,901/month**
- Married: If both are applying, each spouse's income is considered individually, **$2,901/month**

Asset Limit (2025):

- Single: **$2,000**
- Married: **$3,000**

Where to Apply:

- ✅ Apply through your **County Aging & Disability Resource Connection (ADRC)**
- 🌐 www.nj.gov/humanservices/dmahs/home/mltss.html
- 📎 County ADRC contact list: www.state.nj.us/humanservices/doas/home/adrc.html

---

✅ nj familycare (medicaid for duals)

Who It Helps:

- NJ residents with Medicare and very limited income
- Applies to those eligible for both Medicare + Medicaid ("dual eligible")

What It Covers:

- Full Medicaid services including:
  - Dental
  - Vision
  - Non-emergency transportation
- May pay Medicare Part B premium, deductibles, and copays
- Allows access to **Medicare Advantage Dual-Eligible Special Needs Plans (D-SNPs)**

Income Limit (2025):

- Single: **$1,305/month**
- Married: **$1,763/month**

Asset Limit:

- Single: **$4,000**
- Married: **$6,000**

Where to Apply:

- 🌐 https://njfamilycare.dhs.state.nj.us/
- 📞 1-800-701-0710

✅ LIS (Low-Income Subsidy / Extra Help)

Who It Helps:

- Medicare Part D enrollees with limited income
- Especially helpful for those with high prescription drug costs

What It Covers:

- Eliminates Part D deductible
- Lowers or eliminates monthly premium (benchmark plans only)
- Caps copays for generic and brand-name medications
- Protects against late enrollment penalties
- Pay no more than $4.90 for each generic/preferred multi-source drug or biosimilar
- Pay no more than $12.15 for all other drugs
- Once your out-of-pocket costs reaches $2,000, you'll pay $0 for each covered drug

Income Limits (2025, for full LIS):

- Single: **$22,590/year**
- Married: **$30,660/year**

Asset Limits:

- Single: **$17,600**
- Married: **$35,130**

Where to Apply:

- 🌐 www.ssa.gov/extrahelp
- Or call Social Security: 📞 1-800-772-1213
- ✅ If you qualify for QMB, SLMB, or Medicaid — **you may be auto-enrolled**

★ **Important:** If you don't remember applying but notice your prescription copays are consistently low and you're not paying a deductible — **you might already have LIS.** Confirm with Medicare or your plan provider.

📘 glossary + medicare term cheat sheet

If you've made it this far, you've already earned a gold star — but if you ever get lost in Medicare lingo again, this cheat sheet is here to keep you grounded. Use it like a pocket translator.

🔤 a–z of medicare terms

ADRC (Aging and Disability Resource Connection):

Your county's front door for long-term care services like MLTSS. Think of them as the local nerve center for in-home help, adult day programs, and Medicaid waivers.

Annual Election Period (AEP):

October 15–December 7 every year — the window when you can switch drug plans or Medicare Advantage plans.

Assets:

Things you own — bank accounts, stocks, bonds, IRAs, etc. Some programs count them (like QMB), and some don't (like PAAD and Senior Gold).

Benchmark Plan:

A drug plan that meets the cost threshold for programs like LIS and PAAD to cover. Not all plans qualify — if you choose a fancy one, PAAD may not pay the premium.

COBRA:

Temporary coverage from a former employer. Expensive, but sometimes worth keeping while waiting for Medicare to start.

Creditable Coverage:

A health or drug plan that's considered "as good as Medicare." Having this protects you from late enrollment penalties.

Deductible:

What you pay before Medicare or your plan starts covering anything. PAAD and LIS can help eliminate this.

D-SNP (Dual-Eligible Special Needs Plan):

A Medicare Advantage plan built specifically for people who have both Medicare and Medicaid. Often includes dental, vision, and over-the-counter perks.

Extra Help (aka LIS):

A federal program that lowers your prescription drug costs. If you qualify, it cuts your premiums, deductibles, and copays.

Giveback Plan:

A Medicare Advantage plan that refunds part of your Part B premium. Only available if you **don't** have Medicaid or QMB. Can be helpful, but not always the best option.

Lifeline:

State utility assistance — gives you a $225 annual credit toward gas or electric bills. Must qualify for another program (like PAAD or Medicaid) to get it.

LIS (Low-Income Subsidy):

See "Extra Help" above — they're the same thing. Managed by Social Security, often applied automatically if you get QMB, SLMB, or Medicaid.

MLTSS (Managed Long Term Services and Supports):

The program that helps pay for things like home care, transportation, and nursing homes. It's for people who need **hands-on help**, not just financial assistance.

MOOP (Maximum Out-of-Pocket):

The most you'll pay in a year with Medicare Advantage. Once you hit this number, the plan covers 100%. It resets every January.

NJ Save:

The one-stop application for most New Jersey Medicare assistance programs. Fill it out once and you get screened for PAAD, Senior Gold, QMB/SLMB, and Lifeline.

PAAD:

The state's flagship prescription help program. Low copays, no deductible, and help with Part D premiums. Best deal in the building if you qualify.

Part A:

Hospital coverage — think overnight stays, skilled nursing, and hospice. Free if you worked 40+ quarters.

Part B:

Outpatient coverage — doctor visits, specialists, labs, durable medical equipment. This is what that $174.70/month premium goes toward in 2025.

Part C (Medicare Advantage):

An all-in-one private plan that includes Parts A + B and often D. Comes with networks, copays, and perks — but not always the freedom of Original Medicare.

Prescription drug coverage. Can be added to Original Medicare or included in an Advantage plan.

QMB (Qualified Medicare Beneficiary):

Pays your Part B premium **and** your deductibles and copays. If you qualify, your medical bills could drop to almost zero.

SLMB / QI:

Other levels of Medicare Savings Programs. They pay your Part B premium only — but that's still a huge deal if you qualify.

SHIP (State Health Insurance Assistance Program):

Free Medicare help from trained counselors — unbiased, no sales pitch, just information. Every state has one.

Senior Gold:

A backup to PAAD for folks who are over the income limit. Higher copays and a yearly max, but still better than full retail prices.

Social Security Award Letter:

Proof of your income. You'll need it for almost every program.

SSA:

Social Security Administration — the agency that handles your LIS, retirement benefits, and income verification.

resources

Whether you're applying for help, following up on a decision, or just trying to find someone who will answer the phone, this list will give you a solid starting point. Every number, link, and agency below has been verified as active for 2025.

---

nj save application portal

For PAAD, Senior Gold, QMB/SLMB, Lifeline, and general Medicare assistance screening

https://njdoas-ua.force.com/njsave

1-800-792-9745 (NJ Division of Aging Services)

---

nj familycare (medicaid)

For full Medicaid or dual eligibility

https://njfamilycare.dhs.state.nj.us

1-800-701-0710

---

ship (state health insurance assistance program – nj)

Free, unbiased help from trained Medicare counselors

https://www.state.nj.us/humanservices/doas/services/ship/

1-800-792-8820

---

county adrc offices (for mltss and local senior help)

Connects you to home care, long-term support, and more

https://www.state.nj.us/humanservices/doas/home/adrc.html

---

lis / extra help program (federal)

https://www.ssa.gov/extrahelp

Social Security: 1-800-772-1213

---

medicare general help

https://www.medicare.gov

1-800-MEDICARE (1-800-633-4227)

---

discount prescription programs (no insurance required)

- https://www.goodrx.com
- https://www.singlecare.com
- https://www.costplusdrugs.com
- https://www.blinkhealth.com